KIDNEY DETOX BLUEPRINT

YOUR ULTIMATE GUIDE TO CLEANSING AND REVITALIZING YOUR KIDNEYS NATURALLY

TABLE OF CONTENTS

CHAPTER 1

INTRODUCTION: WHY KIDNEY HEALTH MATTERS

1.1 UNDERSTANDING THE ROLE OF THE KIDNEYS

The kidneys are two bean-shaped organs located on either side of your spine, just below the ribcage. Despite their small size, these organs perform a multitude of essential tasks that are vital to keeping your body functioning smoothly.

One of the primary roles of the kidneys is **filtering waste products and toxins** from the blood. They process around 50 gallons of blood daily, removing excess fluids, salts, and waste materials, which are then excreted as urine. This filtration process ensures that harmful substances do not accumulate in the body.

In addition to waste removal, the kidneys play a significant role in maintaining **fluid and electrolyte balance.** They regulate the levels of sodium, potassium, and other minerals in the body, ensuring proper hydration and supporting cellular function.

Another vital function of the kidneys is producing hormones. These hormones regulate essential processes, such as:

Blood pressure control: The kidneys release renin, which helps manage blood pressure by controlling the constriction of blood vessels.

Red blood cell production: Erythropoietin, a hormone produced by the kidneys, stimulates the production of red blood cells in the bone marrow.

Bone health: The kidneys activate vitamin D, a crucial nutrient for calcium absorption and strong bones.

The kidneys' multitasking abilities underscore their importance. When they are not functioning optimally, it can disrupt numerous bodily systems, leading to a cascade of health issues.

1.2 SIGNS AND SYMPTOMS OF KIDNEY STRESS

Despite their resilience, the kidneys can become overworked and stressed, especially when exposed to poor dietary habits, dehydration, medications, and environmental toxins. Identifying early signs of kidney stress is crucial for timely intervention.

Common Symptoms of Kidney Stress:

Fatigue and Low Energy: When the kidneys struggle to remove waste from the blood, toxins can build up, leading to feelings of exhaustion.

Swelling (Edema): The kidneys regulate fluid balance, so impaired function may cause water retention, leading to swelling in the hands, feet, or face.

Frequent or Painful Urination: Changes in urination patterns, such as increased frequency, foamy urine, or discomfort, can indicate kidney stress.

High Blood Pressure: Dysfunctional kidneys can affect blood pressure regulation, often leading to hypertension.

Back Pain or Discomfort: Persistent pain near the lower back or sides could signal underlying kidney issues.

Metallic Taste or Ammonia Breath: A buildup of waste in the bloodstream may alter taste perception or cause bad breath.

Skin Issues: Dry or itchy skin may result from the kidneys' inability to balance minerals and nutrients effectively.

Underlying Causes of Kidney Stress:

Dehydration: Inadequate water intake hinders the kidneys' ability to filter blood efficiently.

High Salt and Sugar Diets: These dietary choices can strain the kidneys, contributing to hypertension and increased workload.

Medications and Toxins: Overuse of certain medications (e.g., painkillers) and exposure to environmental toxins can damage kidney cells over time.

By paying attention to these warning signs, you can take proactive steps to alleviate stress on your kidneys and prevent more severe complications.

1.3 THE BENEFITS OF A KIDNEY DETOX

A kidney detox is a deliberate and natural approach to cleansing and rejuvenating your kidneys. It involves dietary adjustments, increased hydration, and lifestyle changes designed to optimize kidney function and eliminate accumulated toxins.

Key Benefits of a Kidney Detox:

Enhanced Waste Removal: A detox helps your kidneys operate at peak efficiency, flushing out built-up waste and toxins. This process reduces the burden on other organs and improves overall bodily health.

Improved Energy Levels: Removing toxins from your system can combat fatigue and lethargy, leaving you feeling revitalized. Clearer blood circulation ensures that oxygen and nutrients reach your cells more effectively.

Reduced Risk of Kidney Stones: A detox emphasizes hydration and a balanced intake of minerals, which can help prevent the formation of painful kidney stones by dissolving and flushing out mineral deposits.

Lower Blood Pressure: Supporting kidney health improves their ability to regulate blood pressure naturally, potentially reducing the need for medication.

Balanced Fluid Levels: By optimizing hydration, a kidney detox helps prevent water retention and swelling, promoting a healthier balance of fluids in the body.

Stronger Immune Function: A detox strengthens your kidneys' ability to filter out pathogens and harmful substances, bolstering your immune defenses.

Healthier Skin and Hair: Improved kidney function often reflects externally, leading to clearer skin, reduced puffiness, and stronger, shinier hair.

Prevention of Chronic Conditions: A detox can prevent the progression of chronic kidney disease and reduce the risk of related conditions, such as diabetes and cardiovascular disease.

How a Kidney Detox Works: A kidney detox plan typically includes:

Hydration: Drinking plenty of water and herbal teas to flush out toxins.

Dietary Adjustments: Consuming kidney-friendly foods, such as cranberries, watermelon, and leafy greens, while avoiding processed foods, excess salt, and sugar.

Herbs and Supplements: Incorporating natural remedies like dandelion root, parsley, and nettle to support kidney cleansing.

Lifestyle Changes: Engaging in light exercise, reducing stress, and getting adequate sleep to support detoxification processes.

CHAPTER TWO

THE SCIENCE OF KIDNEY DETOXIFICATION

2.1 HOW TOXINS AFFECT KIDNEY FUNCTION

Every day, the human body is exposed to toxins from food, water, air, and even its metabolic processes. While the kidneys are designed to handle these toxins, excessive exposure or prolonged stress can compromise their efficiency.

Types of Toxins That Affect the Kidneys:

Metabolic Waste Products: These are byproducts of cellular metabolism, such as urea and creatinine, that must be excreted to maintain balance.

Dietary Toxins: High-sodium foods, excessive sugar, and processed foods introduce substances that increase the kidneys' workload.

Environmental Toxins: Pollutants, heavy metals (e.g., lead, mercury), and pesticides can accumulate in the bloodstream and harm kidney tissues.

Medications and Substances: Overuse of medications like nonsteroidal anti-inflammatory drugs (NSAIDs), antibiotics, or alcohol can stress or damage kidney cells.

Impact of Toxins on Kidney Health:

Oxidative Stress: Excessive toxins can generate free radicals, molecules that cause damage to kidney cells and tissues through oxidative stress. Over time, this can lead to chronic kidney disease (CKD).

Inflammation: Toxins can trigger inflammatory responses that impair kidney function and disrupt their filtration capabilities.

Kidney Stones: High concentrations of minerals, combined with low hydration, may lead to crystallization, forming painful kidney stones.

Protein Leakage: Damaged kidneys may lose their ability to retain essential proteins like albumin, a condition known as proteinuria.

Chronic Kidney Disease: Persistent exposure to harmful toxins can progressively damage kidney function, potentially leading to kidney failure.

A build-up of toxins not only weakens the kidneys but also affects other bodily systems, as the waste they are meant to remove lingers in the bloodstream. Understanding how these substances affect kidney function underscores the need for regular detoxification.

2.2 KEY DETOXIFICATION PROCESSES

The kidneys rely on a series of intricate processes to filter the blood, remove toxins, and maintain homeostasis. Supporting these processes through detox strategies enhances kidney efficiency.

Key Steps in Kidney Detoxification:

Filtration:

Blood enters the kidneys through the renal arteries, where

millions of microscopic structures called nephrons perform the filtration process. Each nephron contains a glomerulus, a tiny filter that removes waste, toxins, and excess water from the blood. This filtered fluid, now called filtrate, moves to the next stage for further processing.

Reabsorption:

The kidneys are highly efficient, reabsorbing vital substances such as glucose, electrolytes, and water back into the bloodstream. This ensures the body retains necessary nutrients while discarding harmful substances.

Secretion:

Additional toxins, hydrogen ions, and waste products that were not filtered out during the initial process are secreted into the filtrate at this stage. This step fine-tunes the body's chemical balance.

Excretion:

Finally, the processed filtrate, now called urine, is transported to the bladder and excreted from the body. This urine carries toxins, waste products, and excess substances out of the body, completing the detoxification process.

Supportive Mechanisms for Kidney Detoxification:

Acid-Base Regulation: The kidneys regulate the body's pH by excreting hydrogen ions and reabsorbing bicarbonate, ensuring an optimal environment for metabolic processes.

Electrolyte Balance: Maintaining appropriate levels of sodium, potassium, and calcium is essential for hydration, nerve function, and muscle contractions.

Hormonal Production: Hormones like erythropoietin and renin, produced by the kidneys, play a role in oxygen delivery and blood pressure regulation, indirectly supporting detoxification.

By promoting these processes through dietary and lifestyle changes, the kidneys can work more efficiently to eliminate harmful substances and sustain overall health.

2.3 THE IMPORTANCE OF HYDRATION

Hydration is arguably the cornerstone of kidney health and detoxification. The kidneys depend on an adequate water supply to perform their functions effectively. Without sufficient hydration, the entire detoxification process becomes compromised.

How Hydration Supports Kidney Function:

Dilution of Urine: Water helps dilute urine, preventing the concentration of waste products and reducing the risk of kidney stones and infections.

Facilitation of Filtration: Blood must remain fluid for optimal circulation through the kidneys. Dehydration thickens blood, making filtration more difficult and less effective.

Toxin Removal: Adequate water intake ensures the kidneys can efficiently flush out toxins, reducing the risk of buildup and related complications.

Temperature Regulation: Water supports thermoregulation, indirectly protecting kidney tissues from the stress of overheating.

Signs of Dehydration That Impact Kidney Health:

- Dark-colored urine
- Reduced urination frequency
- Dry skin and mucous membranes
- Fatigue and dizziness
- Muscle cramps

Optimal Hydration Practices for Kidney Detox:

Drink Plenty of Water: Aim for at least 8-10 glasses (2-3 liters) daily, adjusting for activity level, climate, and individual needs.

Incorporate Herbal Teas: Herbal teas like nettle, dandelion, and parsley have diuretic properties that support kidney detox.

Limit Sugary or Caffeinated Beverages: These can dehydrate the body and place additional stress on the kidneys.

Consume Water-Rich Foods: Foods like watermelon, cucumber, and celery can supplement water intake while providing essential nutrients.

The Risks of Chronic Dehydration: Long-term dehydration can lead to a host of kidney-related problems, including the formation of stones, urinary tract infections, and impaired waste filtration. In severe cases, chronic dehydration can contribute to kidney damage and disease progression.

CHAPTER THREE

FOODS THAT SUPPORT KIDNEY HEALTH

3.1 TOP KIDNEY-FRIENDLY SUPERFOODS

Certain foods are particularly beneficial for supporting kidney health. These superfoods are nutrient-rich, promote detoxification, and help reduce the risk of kidney-related issues.

1. Cranberries: Cranberries are renowned for their role in preventing urinary tract infections (UTIs), which can harm the kidneys if left untreated. Rich in antioxidants and proanthocyanidins, cranberries reduce bacteria adhesion to the urinary tract lining and support kidney health.

2. Blueberries: Blueberries are packed with antioxidants like anthocyanins, which help reduce inflammation and protect kidney cells from oxidative stress. They are also low in potassium, making them ideal for kidney health.

3. Garlic: Garlic is a natural anti-inflammatory and antioxidant powerhouse. It helps lower cholesterol levels, reduce blood pressure, and combat toxins that can damage the kidneys.

4. Red Bell Peppers: Red bell peppers are low in potassium but high in essential nutrients like vitamin C, vitamin A, and folic acid. They support kidney function and overall health.

5. Cabbage: Cabbage is a cruciferous vegetable that provides vitamins K, C, and B6, along with fiber. It promotes digestion and helps the kidneys eliminate waste more effectively.

6. Apples: Rich in fiber and anti-inflammatory compounds, apples support kidney health by improving digestion and reducing cholesterol levels. They also help regulate blood sugar, which is critical for preventing kidney damage in diabetic individuals.

7. Onions: Onions are low in potassium and contain quercetin, a potent antioxidant that fights inflammation. They are an excellent addition to kidney-friendly diets.

8. Watermelon: Watermelon is hydrating and contains lycopene, an antioxidant that supports kidney health by reducing oxidative stress. Its high water content aids in flushing out toxins.

9. Pumpkin Seeds: Pumpkin seeds provide magnesium and other essential minerals that support overall kidney function. Consuming them in moderation can help prevent kidney stones.

10. Parsley: Parsley is a natural diuretic that helps flush out toxins and excess fluid. It can also reduce the risk of kidney stone formation.

Incorporating these superfoods into your meals ensures that your kidneys receive the nutrients they need to function optimally.

3.2 FOODS TO AVOID DURING DETOX

While focusing on kidney-friendly foods, it's equally important to avoid foods that can strain or harm the kidneys during a detox. Certain dietary choices can increase the workload on the kidneys, disrupt their balance, or lead to toxin buildup.

1. Processed Foods: Highly processed foods, such as chips, canned soups, and fast food, often contain excessive amounts of sodium and preservatives. These can lead to water retention and elevate blood pressure, putting stress on the kidneys.

2. High-Sugar Foods: Excessive sugar intake can lead to weight gain, insulin resistance, and diabetes, all of which increase the risk of kidney damage. Avoid sugary drinks, candies, and desserts during a detox.

3. Red and Processed Meats: Red meat and processed meats like sausages and deli cuts are high in protein and saturated fat, which can burden the kidneys. During detox, opt for plant-based proteins or lean meats.

4. Dairy Products: Dairy products, such as cheese, milk, and cream, are high in phosphorus and potassium, which can disrupt mineral balance in people with compromised kidney function.

5. High-Oxalate Foods: Foods like spinach, beets, and rhubarb contain high levels of oxalates, which can contribute to kidney stone formation. Limit these during a detox.

6. Alcohol: Alcohol is a toxin that dehydrates the body and impairs kidney function. It's best to avoid alcohol completely during a kidney detox.

7. Caffeine: Excessive caffeine from coffee, tea, and energy drinks can increase blood pressure and stress the kidneys. Moderation is key, or consider caffeine-free alternatives during detox.

8. Salty Snacks: Chips, salted nuts, and crackers are loaded with sodium, which can lead to fluid retention and high blood pressure. Choose unsalted or lightly seasoned snacks instead.

By avoiding these foods, you reduce the burden on your kidneys, allowing them to focus on detoxification and repair.

3.3 RECIPES FOR A KIDNEY-CLEANSING DIET

Incorporating kidney-friendly superfoods into delicious recipes can make detoxing enjoyable and sustainable. Below are three simple, nutrient-packed recipes designed to support kidney health.

Recipe 1: Cranberry & Apple Detox Smoothie
Ingredients:

- 1 cup unsweetened cranberry juice
- 1 medium apple (chopped)
- ½ cup blueberries
- 1 tablespoon lemon juice
- 1 cup water or coconut water
- Ice cubes (optional)

Instructions:

1. Combine all ingredients in a blender.
2. Blend until smooth.
3. Serve chilled and enjoy a refreshing detox boost.

Benefits: This smoothie is packed with antioxidants, vitamin C, and hydration to support kidney detoxification.

Recipe 2: Garlic & Parsley Quinoa Salad

Ingredients:

- 1 cup cooked quinoa
- 2 cloves garlic (minced)
- 1 cup fresh parsley (chopped)
- 1 red bell pepper (diced)
- 2 tablespoons olive oil

- 1 tablespoon lemon juice
- Salt and pepper to taste

Instructions:

1. In a large bowl, mix cooked quinoa, garlic, parsley, and red bell pepper.
2. Drizzle with olive oil and lemon juice.
3. Season with salt and pepper to taste.
4. Toss well and serve as a light, kidney-friendly meal.

Benefits: This dish combines low-potassium ingredients with detoxifying herbs to promote kidney health.

Recipe 3: Watermelon & Mint Hydration Salad

Ingredients:

- 2 cups watermelon (cubed)
- ¼ cup fresh mint leaves
- 1 tablespoon lime juice
- 1 teaspoon honey (optional)

Instructions:

1. In a bowl, combine watermelon and mint leaves.

2. Drizzle with lime juice and honey if desired.

3. Chill before serving for a hydrating snack or side dish.

Benefits: High water content and antioxidants make this salad a perfect addition to a kidney-cleansing diet.

CHAPTER FOUR

HERBS AND NATURAL REMEDIES FOR KIDNEY DETOX

4.1 POWERFUL HERBS FOR CLEANSING

Herbs have been used for centuries in traditional medicine to cleanse and rejuvenate the kidneys. These plants are packed with bioactive compounds that support detoxification and reduce the risk of kidney-related ailments.

1. Dandelion Root: Dandelion root acts as a natural diuretic, helping the kidneys eliminate excess water and toxins. It's also rich in antioxidants that reduce oxidative stress on kidney cells.

How to Use:

Brew dandelion root tea by steeping 1–2 teaspoons of dried root in boiling water for 10 minutes. Drink daily for optimal results.

2. Nettle Leaf: Nettle leaf is a nutrient-dense herb that promotes increased urine production, flushing out waste and supporting kidney function. It also has anti-inflammatory properties.

How to Use:

Add nettle leaf to soups or stews, or prepare as a tea. Drink 1–2 cups per day during a detox.

3. Parsley: Parsley is a natural diuretic that encourages the elimination of toxins. Its high levels of vitamins A and C also support overall kidney health.

How to Use:

Blend fresh parsley into smoothies, use it in salads, or steep the leaves in hot water for a refreshing tea.

4. Marshmallow Root: Marshmallow root soothes the urinary tract, reducing inflammation and promoting healthy kidney function. Its mucilage content provides a protective coating to tissues.

How to Use:

Steep 1–2 teaspoons of dried marshmallow root in cold water overnight. Strain and drink the infusion in the morning.

5. Turmeric: Turmeric is a powerful anti-inflammatory and antioxidant herb that protects the kidneys from damage. It also supports the liver, aiding overall detoxification.

How to Use:

Add turmeric powder to curries, golden milk, or smoothies, or take it as a supplement.

6. Ginger: Ginger improves circulation and reduces inflammation, making it an excellent herb for supporting kidney health and boosting detox processes.

How to Use:

Brew ginger tea by simmering fresh slices in water for 10 minutes, or incorporate ginger into your meals and smoothies.

7. Burdock Root: Burdock root has detoxifying properties that help the kidneys and liver remove harmful substances. It also supports the body's natural filtration systems.

How to Use:

Add burdock root to soups or teas for a gentle detox boost.

Using these herbs regularly can naturally enhance your kidneys' ability to cleanse and maintain balance.

4.2 SUPPLEMENTS TO BOOST KIDNEY FUNCTION

In addition to herbs, certain supplements can help improve kidney function and support overall health during a detox. These supplements are typically derived from natural sources and target specific aspects of kidney performance.

1. Cranberry Extract: Cranberry supplements contain concentrated antioxidants that prevent bacteria from adhering to the urinary tract lining, reducing the risk of infections and supporting kidney function.

Recommended Dosage:

Take 300–400 mg daily, or as directed on the product label.

2. Magnesium: Magnesium helps prevent the formation of kidney stones by regulating calcium and oxalate levels in the body.

Recommended Dosage:

Adults typically need 310–420 mg per day, depending on age and gender.

3. Vitamin B6: Vitamin B6 supports protein metabolism and prevents excessive oxalate buildup, which can lead to kidney stones.

Recommended Dosage:

1.3–2 mg per day, as part of a balanced diet or a multivitamin.

4. Omega-3 Fatty Acids: Found in fish oil or flaxseed oil, omega-3 fatty acids reduce inflammation and support the overall health of kidney tissues.

Recommended Dosage:

1,000–2,000 mg of EPA and DHA combined per day.

5. Probiotics: Probiotics balance gut bacteria, which indirectly supports kidney health by reducing the production of harmful toxins that kidneys must filter.

Recommended Dosage:

Take a probiotic supplement with at least 10 billion CFUs daily.

6. Milk Thistle: Milk thistle supports the liver in detoxification processes, which indirectly benefits the kidneys by reducing their workload.

Recommended Dosage:

200–400 mg of standardized extract per day.

When using supplements, it's essential to follow recommended dosages and consult with a healthcare professional, especially if you have pre-existing health conditions or are on medications.

4.3 DIY HERBAL TEAS AND REMEDIES

Incorporating herbal teas and natural remedies into your daily routine is a simple and effective way to support kidney detoxification. Here are some easy-to-make remedies:

1. Kidney Detox Herbal Tea Blend Ingredients:

- 1 teaspoon dried dandelion root
- 1 teaspoon dried nettle leaf
- 1 teaspoon parsley flakes
- 2 cups boiling water

Instructions:

1. Combine the herbs in a teapot or strainer.
2. Pour boiling water over the herbs and steep for 10 minutes.
3. Strain and enjoy.

Benefits: This tea promotes diuresis, flushing out toxins, and providing essential nutrients for kidney health.

---

2. Ginger-Turmeric Detox Shot

Ingredients:

- 1 teaspoon fresh ginger juice
- 1 teaspoon turmeric powder
- Juice of 1 lemon
- 1 cup water

Instructions:

1. Mix all ingredients in a small glass.

2. Drink first thing in the morning for a detoxifying boost.

Benefits: This shot reduces inflammation, improves circulation, and supports kidney cleansing.

---

3. Parsley and Lemon Juice Tonic

Ingredients:

- 1 cup fresh parsley leaves
- Juice of 1 lemon
- 1 cup water

Instructions:

1. Blend parsley leaves and water until smooth.
2. Strain and mix with lemon juice.
3. Drink immediately.

Benefits: This tonic aids in flushing out toxins and provides a refreshing, nutrient-packed boost.

---

4. Soothing Marshmallow Root Infusion

Ingredients:

- 2 tablespoons dried marshmallow root
- 2 cups cold water

Instructions:

1. Add marshmallow root to a jar and cover with cold water.
2. Let it sit overnight (8–12 hours).
3. Strain and drink throughout the day.

Benefits: This infusion soothes the urinary tract and reduces inflammation.

By incorporating these herbs, supplements, and remedies into your kidney detox plan, you can naturally enhance your body's ability to cleanse and rejuvenate. These practices are not only effective but also simple to implement, making them an excellent addition to a healthier lifestyle.

CHAPTER FIVE

LIFESTYLE PRACTICES TO ENHANCE KIDNEY
DETOX

5.1 THE ROLE OF EXERCISE IN KIDNEY HEALTH

Exercise is a cornerstone of a healthy lifestyle and has a profound impact on kidney function. Regular physical activity promotes cardiovascular health, enhances circulation, and supports detoxification processes.

1. Improving Blood Flow to the Kidneys: The kidneys rely on a steady supply of oxygen-rich blood to filter toxins effectively. Exercise increases blood circulation, ensuring that the kidneys receive the nutrients and oxygen they need to function optimally. Improved circulation also aids in the removal of waste products from the body.

2. Regulating Blood Pressure: High blood pressure is one of the leading causes of kidney damage. Regular physical activity helps regulate blood pressure by strengthening the heart and improving arterial health. Activities like walking, swimming, and cycling are particularly beneficial for maintaining healthy blood pressure levels.

3. Enhancing Toxin Elimination: Exercise encourages sweating, another pathway for toxin elimination. As sweat glands expel waste products, the kidneys experience a reduced burden, allowing them to focus on other vital functions.

4. Reducing the Risk of Chronic Kidney Disease (CKD): Studies have shown that maintaining an active lifestyle lowers the risk of developing CKD. Physical activity reduces inflammation, supports weight management, and improves insulin sensitivity, all of which contribute to kidney health.

Exercise Recommendations for Kidney Health:

Aerobic Exercise: Engage in moderate aerobic activities like brisk walking, jogging, or dancing for at least 150 minutes per week.

Strength Training: Incorporate strength exercises 2–3 times per week to maintain muscle mass and support overall metabolic health.

Stretching and Yoga: These practices improve flexibility, circulation, and stress management, indirectly benefiting the kidneys.

By making exercise a regular part of your routine, you can enhance detoxification processes and support the long-term health of your kidneys.

5.2 STRESS REDUCTION AND ITS IMPACT ON DETOXIFICATION

Stress has a significant influence on kidney function and overall health. Chronic stress triggers a cascade of physiological responses that can impair detoxification processes and damage the kidneys over time.

1. The Stress-Kidney Connection: When you experience stress, your body releases hormones like cortisol and adrenaline. While these hormones are helpful in short-term situations, chronic stress leads to elevated blood pressure and increased blood sugar levels—both of which strain the kidneys.

2. Impact on Kidney Function

- **Elevated Blood Pressure:** Prolonged stress can lead to hypertension, a primary risk factor for kidney disease.

- **Increased Inflammation:** Chronic stress promotes inflammation, which can damage kidney tissues and impair filtration.
- **Hormonal Imbalance:** Stress disrupts the delicate hormonal balance necessary for proper kidney function, including the regulation of fluid and electrolyte levels.

3. Stress Reduction Techniques: Adopting stress management practices can significantly enhance kidney detoxification and overall health:

- **Meditation and Mindfulness:** Practices like meditation and mindfulness reduce cortisol levels, promote relaxation, and support kidney function. Even 10 minutes of daily meditation can make a difference.
- **Deep Breathing Exercises:** Breathing exercises calm the nervous system, lower blood pressure, and improve circulation. Try diaphragmatic breathing for a simple yet effective stress-relief technique.
- **Yoga:** Combining physical movement with breath control, yoga helps reduce stress while promoting flexibility and circulation.
- **Nature Walks:** Spending time in nature has been shown to lower stress hormones and improve overall well-being.

By actively managing stress, you create an environment in which your kidneys can perform their detoxifying roles without interference.

5.3 SLEEP AND KIDNEY REPAIR

Sleep is a vital component of health, providing the body with the time it needs to repair and rejuvenate. For the kidneys, sleep is a critical period for detoxification, regulation, and restoration.

1. The Role of Sleep in Kidney Health: During sleep, the body undergoes numerous processes that support kidney function:

- **Toxin Removal:** The kidneys continue filtering blood during sleep, working to remove waste products and toxins that accumulate throughout the day.
- **Hormonal Regulation:** Sleep supports the balance of hormones like vasopressin, which helps regulate the body's water levels and kidney function.
- **Repair and Regeneration:** Sleep allows kidney cells to repair damage caused by daily wear and tear, oxidative stress, and toxin exposure.

2. Consequences of Poor Sleep on Kidney Health: Inadequate sleep, whether due to insomnia, sleep apnea, or poor sleep hygiene, can have detrimental effects on the kidneys:

- **Increased Blood Pressure:** Sleep deprivation leads to elevated blood pressure, a significant risk factor for kidney disease.
- **Reduced Filtration Efficiency:** Lack of sleep impairs the kidneys' ability to filter waste effectively, leading to toxin buildup.
- **Chronic Kidney Damage:** Over time, poor sleep quality is associated with an increased risk of CKD and kidney failure.

3. Tips for Enhancing Sleep Quality: To support kidney health, prioritize restorative sleep by adopting these habits:

- **Establish a Sleep Schedule:** Go to bed and wake up at the same time each day to regulate your circadian rhythm.
- **Create a Sleep-Friendly Environment:** Ensure your bedroom is dark, quiet, and cool, with a comfortable mattress and bedding.

- **Limit Screen Time:** Avoid screens at least an hour before bedtime, as the blue light emitted can disrupt melatonin production.
- **Avoid Stimulants:** Refrain from consuming caffeine, nicotine, or heavy meals in the hours leading up to bedtime.
- **Practice Relaxation Techniques:** Wind down with activities like reading, gentle yoga, or a warm bath before bed.

4. The Importance of Consistent Sleep Patterns: Consistently getting 7–9 hours of sleep per night allows your kidneys to perform their detoxification and repair processes efficiently. Sleep is not just rest—it's an active period of healing that is essential for your overall health.

CHAPTER SIX

THE 7-DAY KIDNEY DETOX PLAN

6.1 DAILY DETOX GOALS AND ACTIVITIES

Each day of the kidney detox plan focuses on specific activities to cleanse the kidneys, promote overall detoxification, and create sustainable habits.

Day 1: Hydration and Preparation

Goal: Start your detox by prioritizing hydration and preparing your body and mind.

Activities:

- Drink at least 2 liters of filtered water throughout the day.
- Eliminate processed foods, caffeine, and alcohol from your diet.
- Begin incorporating kidney-friendly herbs like dandelion root tea.

Day 2: Nourish with Kidney-Supporting Foods

Goal: Introduce nutrient-dense, kidney-friendly foods into your diet.

Activities:

- Focus on fresh fruits and vegetables like watermelon, cucumbers, and leafy greens.
- Enjoy a simple salad with parsley and lemon dressing for lunch.
- Prepare steamed asparagus or sweet potatoes for dinner.

Day 3: Move for Detox

Goal: Engage in gentle exercise to boost circulation and toxin elimination.

Activities:

- Begin your day with a 20-minute brisk walk or yoga session.
- Continue hydrating with water infused with cucumber and mint.
- Incorporate a ginger-turmeric shot in the morning to reduce inflammation.

Day 4: Herbal Support and Relaxation

Goal: Use herbal teas and relaxation techniques to support kidney function.

Activities:

- Sip nettle leaf tea in the morning and marshmallow root tea in the evening.
- Practice mindfulness meditation for 10 minutes to reduce stress.
- Include a kidney-cleansing smoothie with berries and spinach for breakfast.

Day 5: Deep Detox with Nutrient Boosts

Goal: Provide your body with extra nutrients for optimal kidney function.

Activities:

- Start your day with a warm glass of lemon water.
- Incorporate potassium-rich foods like bananas and avocados into your meals.
- Take a relaxing Epsom salt bath in the evening to encourage toxin release.

Day 6: Renew and Recharge

Goal: Continue supporting kidney health with balanced meals and hydration.

Activities:

- Drink 3 cups of herbal tea spread throughout the day.
- Focus on whole grains like quinoa and kidney-friendly proteins like lentils.
- Spend time in nature to boost mental and physical well-being.

Day 7: Reflection and Long-Term Planning

Goal: Conclude your detox with a plan to maintain healthy habits.

Activities:

- Reflect on your progress and write down any changes you've noticed.
- Create a long-term meal and lifestyle plan to support ongoing kidney health.
- Celebrate your success with a nourishing, balanced dinner.

6.2 MEAL PLANS AND HYDRATION TIPS

Eating the right foods and staying properly hydrated are foundational to a successful kidney detox. This section provides meal ideas and hydration strategies to fuel your detox journey.

Sample Daily Meal Plan

Breakfast:

- **Green Smoothie:** Blend spinach, cucumber, parsley, lemon juice, and a handful of frozen berries with coconut water.
- **Herbal Tea:** Start your day with dandelion root tea to kickstart detoxification.

Mid-Morning Snack:

- **Fruit Plate:** Enjoy a mix of watermelon, cantaloupe, and apple slices.
- **Hydration:** Sip on water infused with mint and lime.

Lunch:

- **Kidney-Friendly Salad:** Combine arugula, cherry tomatoes, steamed asparagus, and a sprinkle of sunflower seeds. Dress with olive oil and lemon juice.
- **Side:** A small serving of quinoa for added protein and fiber.

Afternoon Snack:

- **Smoothie Bowl:** Blend a frozen banana with almond milk, top with chia seeds and fresh blueberries.

Dinner:

- **Grilled Salmon or Tofu:** Pair with steamed broccoli and a baked sweet potato.
- **Hydration:** Drink nettle tea to enhance kidney function before bed.

Hydration Tips for Maximum Effectiveness
Proper hydration is crucial during a kidney detox. Here's how to ensure your body gets the fluids it needs:

1. **Drink Consistently:** Aim for 2–3 liters of water daily, spread evenly throughout the day.

2. **Enhance Your Water:** Add slices of cucumber, lemon, or ginger to improve flavor and provide additional detox benefits.

3. **Incorporate Herbal Teas:** Sip teas like nettle, parsley, or marshmallow root for hydration and added kidney support.

4. **Avoid Dehydrators:** Steer clear of caffeine, alcohol, and sugary drinks, as they can strain the kidneys.

By following these meal plans and hydration guidelines, you can nourish your body and support efficient detoxification.

6.3 TRACKING YOUR PROGRESS

Monitoring your progress is essential to staying motivated and identifying the positive changes in your body during the detox.

Why Track Your Progress?
Tracking helps you:

- Measure improvements in energy levels, mood, and physical health.

- Identify any foods or habits that don't align with your detox goals.
- Celebrate small victories to stay motivated.

Tools for Tracking:

1. **Journal:** Dedicate a notebook to your kidney detox journey. Write down your meals, water intake, and any observations about how you feel.
2. **Apps:** Use health-tracking apps to monitor hydration, exercise, and mood changes.
3. **Photos:** Take before-and-after photos to visually document improvements, like reduced bloating or clearer skin.

What to Track:

- **Physical Changes:** Note improvements in energy levels, digestion, and any reduction in bloating or water retention.
- **Mental Well-Being:** Record changes in mood, stress levels, and sleep quality.
- **Kidney-Specific Benefits:** Pay attention to any changes in urinary patterns or overall comfort in the abdominal area.

Daily Reflection Questions:

- Did I meet my hydration goal today?
- How did my body feel after meals?
- Did I incorporate exercise or stress-reduction techniques?
- What improvements have I noticed since starting the detox?

Staying Accountable:

- Share your progress with a friend or family member for encouragement.
- Reward yourself for completing each day's goals—non-food rewards like a relaxing bath or a new book are great options.

CHAPTER SEVEN

MAINTAINING KIDNEY HEALTH LONG-TERM

7.1 POST-DETOX BEST PRACTICES

After completing a kidney detox, your body is in a refreshed and balanced state. Maintaining this momentum is key to reaping the long-term benefits. First, focus on continuing a diet rich in kidney-supporting foods. Leafy greens, berries, citrus fruits, and whole grains should remain staples in your meals, as they help maintain the detoxified state of your kidneys. Avoid falling back into the habit of consuming processed foods, sugary drinks, and excessive sodium, as these can reverse the progress you've made.

Hydration should also remain a priority. Drinking enough water is not just for detox periods—it is a lifelong practice that ensures the kidneys can filter waste and toxins effectively. Incorporate herbal teas like nettle, parsley, or dandelion root into your daily routine, as they provide a gentle, natural way to continue supporting kidney function.

Physical activity, even in moderation, also contributes significantly to maintaining kidney health. Gentle exercises like walking, yoga, or swimming encourage healthy blood circulation and reduce the risk of conditions such as high blood pressure, which can harm the kidneys over time. Aim to stay active daily, even if it's just a short walk during your lunch break or a few stretches in the morning.

Stress management is equally essential in preserving the benefits of your kidney detox. Chronic stress can lead to elevated blood pressure and inflammation, which negatively impact kidney function. Make relaxation practices, such as mindfulness meditation or deep breathing exercises, part of your routine. Even dedicating 10 minutes a day to stress relief can have profound effects on your mental and physical health.

7.2 HOW TO PREVENT KIDNEY ISSUES IN THE FUTURE

Preventing kidney-related problems requires a proactive approach. Begin by understanding the key risk factors, such as high blood pressure, diabetes, obesity, and a family history of kidney disease. Awareness of these risks enables you to take preventive measures and monitor your health closely.

One of the most effective ways to safeguard your kidneys is through mindful nutrition. Limit your intake of sodium, as excessive salt can strain the kidneys and lead to high blood pressure. Season your meals with herbs and spices instead of relying on salt to enhance flavor. Additionally, monitor your protein intake. While protein is essential for the body, consuming it in excess—especially from animal sources—can burden the kidneys over time. Opt for plant-based protein sources like lentils, chickpeas, and tofu to reduce this strain.

Another vital aspect of prevention is regular checkups. Schedule routine blood pressure and glucose tests to detect any early signs of hypertension or diabetes. Both conditions are leading causes of kidney damage, but they can often be managed effectively when caught early. If you have a history of kidney issues or other risk factors, discuss regular kidney function tests with your healthcare provider to ensure any problems are addressed promptly.

Avoiding harmful substances also plays a significant role in kidney health. Minimize your consumption of alcohol, and avoid smoking, as both can lead to kidney damage and other health complications. Over-the-counter pain relievers, such as ibuprofen and aspirin, should also be used sparingly, as prolonged use can harm the kidneys. Always consult a healthcare professional before taking any medication or supplement, particularly if you have existing kidney concerns.

Physical activity and weight management are additional pillars of kidney health. Maintaining a healthy weight reduces the risk of diabetes and high blood pressure, which are closely linked to kidney issues. Regular exercise not only helps manage weight but also boosts circulation, reduces inflammation, and supports the body's detoxification processes.

Lastly, prioritize sleep. Poor sleep has been linked to a decline in kidney function, as the body's repair and regulatory processes are disrupted. Aim for 7–9 hours of quality sleep per night by creating a bedtime routine and maintaining a consistent sleep schedule.

7.3 INTEGRATING DETOX HABITS INTO YOUR DAILY LIFE

Sustaining the benefits of a kidney detox doesn't mean living in a constant state of restriction. Instead, the key is to weave detox practices into your everyday routine in a way that feels natural and enjoyable.

Begin by making small but meaningful dietary adjustments. For instance, start each day with a glass of warm lemon water to hydrate your body and support kidney function. Replace one meal a week with a kidney-friendly smoothie made from spinach, cucumber, parsley, and berries. Gradually increasing the presence of these nutrient-dense foods in your diet will create lasting habits without overwhelming your routine.

Hydration can also be a consistent, effortless habit. Carry a reusable water bottle wherever you go to remind yourself to drink regularly. Experiment with infused waters by adding slices of citrus, ginger, or fresh herbs for a refreshing twist. Staying hydrated is one of the simplest ways to protect your kidneys and support detoxification.

Incorporate movement into your day, even if you have a busy schedule. Simple changes like taking the stairs, parking farther from your destination, or setting a timer for hourly stretch breaks can make a big difference over time. If you enjoy structure, commit to a weekly yoga or Pilates class, which supports kidney health through enhanced circulation and stress relief.

Detoxification doesn't have to be limited to physical habits—consider incorporating mental detox practices as well. Dedicate time each week to reflect, journal, or meditate, allowing your mind to release stress and tension. A balanced mental state positively impacts your physical health, including your kidneys.

Regularly prepare herbal teas that promote kidney health, such as nettle or dandelion root tea, and enjoy them as part of your evening routine. These small rituals not only benefit your kidneys but also provide moments of relaxation and mindfulness.

Set realistic, long-term goals for maintaining your kidney health. For example, aim to gradually reduce processed food consumption over several months or commit to trying a new kidney-friendly recipe each week. Celebrate your achievements, no matter how small, as they contribute to a healthier lifestyle.

Integrating detox habits into your daily life is about balance and consistency rather than perfection. By adopting these practices gradually, you can sustain the benefits of a kidney detox while enjoying a vibrant, healthy life.

CHAPTER EIGHT

CONCLUSION: A JOURNEY TO LIFELONG KIDNEY WELLNESS

As you reach the end of your kidney detox journey, it's important to reflect on the strides you've made, the lessons you've learned, and the habits you've cultivated. This isn't merely the conclusion of a week-long effort to cleanse and revitalize your kidneys; it's the beginning of a lifelong commitment to your health and well-being. The path to maintaining vibrant kidney health is one of continuous care, mindfulness, and empowerment, and it's a journey that can transform not only your physical health but also your mental and emotional resilience.

8.1 REFLECTING ON YOUR DETOX JOURNEY

Reflecting on the process of detoxification is a powerful way to acknowledge the work you've done and understand its impact on your body and mind. Over the past few days or weeks, you've likely experienced a range of physical changes. Perhaps you've noticed a boost in energy levels, clearer skin, or an improved sense of well-being. These positive changes are a testament to the body's incredible ability to heal and renew itself when given the proper support.

Equally significant are the shifts in mindset that often accompany a detox journey. Choosing to care for your kidneys and prioritizing their health represents a decision to take control of your overall wellness. This empowerment extends beyond the physical realm; it influences how you approach challenges, make decisions, and set goals in all areas of your life. Reflecting on this experience allows you to celebrate the victories—both large and small—that have brought you to this point.

Remember that reflection isn't just about acknowledging successes; it's also an opportunity to identify areas for growth. Were there moments when you struggled to stay consistent with your detox plan? Did you encounter obstacles that made certain aspects of the process challenging? By examining these experiences without judgment, you can better prepare for the future, equipping yourself with strategies to navigate similar situations more effectively.

8.2 STAYING COMMITTED TO YOUR HEALTH GOALS

Staying committed to your health goals is a natural extension of the progress you've made during this detox journey. The habits and practices you've developed—whether it's drinking more water, incorporating kidney-friendly foods into your diet, or finding time for stress relief—are building blocks for a healthier, more balanced lifestyle. It's essential to maintain this momentum and keep your goals in focus as you move forward.

Commitment often requires a shift in perspective. Instead of viewing kidney health as a temporary project, embrace it as an integral part of your daily life. Think of the small, consistent actions you take—such as choosing whole, unprocessed foods or prioritizing sleep—not as chores, but as gifts you give yourself. This mindset transforms healthy living into a source of joy and self-respect rather than an obligation.

To stay motivated, consider setting specific, measurable, and realistic goals for the future. For example, you might aim to drink a certain amount of water each day, exercise three times a week, or prepare one kidney-friendly recipe every weekend. Tracking your progress, whether through a journal, an app, or even simple checklists, can help you stay accountable and celebrate your achievements along the way.

Community support can also play a significant role in maintaining your commitment. Sharing your goals with friends, family, or a like-minded group creates a network of encouragement and accountability. Whether it's swapping healthy recipes, joining a fitness class, or participating in discussions about wellness, these connections reinforce your dedication and provide inspiration to keep going.

There will inevitably be days when staying committed feels challenging, and that's okay. Life is full of fluctuations, and it's important to approach these moments with compassion rather than criticism. Remind yourself of your "why"—the reasons you began this journey—and use that motivation to recalibrate and refocus. Progress isn't about perfection; it's about persistence.

8.3 FINAL WORDS OF ENCOURAGEMENT

As you move forward, carry with you the understanding that kidney health is deeply connected to your overall well-being. The practices you've adopted during this detox don't just benefit your kidneys; they positively impact your entire body and mind. Every step you take toward better health—no matter how small—contributes to a stronger, more vibrant version of yourself.

Remember that the journey to lifelong kidney wellness is a personal one. While general guidelines and recommendations are valuable, your path will be unique, shaped by your individual needs, preferences, and circumstances. Listen to your body, trust your instincts, and make adjustments as needed.

Finally, take pride in the fact that you've chosen to prioritize your health. In a world filled with distractions and demands, committing to self-care is a powerful act of resilience and self-love. Your dedication to improving and maintaining your kidney health sets a foundation for a life of vitality, balance, and happiness.

In closing, let this chapter serve as a reminder of the incredible strength and potential within you. You have the tools, knowledge, and determination to care for your kidneys and your overall health for years to come. Embrace this journey with curiosity and compassion, and know that every effort you make is a step toward a brighter, healthier future.

Your kidneys are essential allies in your body's intricate symphony of life, and by caring for them, you honor the gift of health and the extraordinary capabilities of your body. Celebrate this journey, continue learning, and most importantly, cherish the sense of well-being that comes from nurturing yourself. Here's to lifelong kidney wellness and a vibrant, fulfilling life ahead.